5 Steps to Helping a Loved One with Mental Illness

Untold Stories Global, LLC
info@untoldstoriesglobal.com

ISBN-13: 978-0-0075546-1-8

5 Steps to Helping a Loved One with Mental Illness

(Bringing Awareness and Support to Families and Communities)

When I first started writing this book, I understood the importance and the impact that it would have on families. As a result of being a mental health advocate I have seen families torn apart for their lack of understanding and of knowledge concerning mental illness. The hopes with this book is to bring families closer together by providing them with some tools and information that would help them be a support to their loved ones and for them to find the support that is needed for themselves.

There are more Americans who experience some form of mental illness then they care to share and or express. As a result, many people have had suicidal thoughts and have completed suicide without family members knowing anything was ever wrong. In recent years we have seen more celebrities come forward to talk about their bouts with mental illness and encourage others to get help.

This book is written by someone who is not only a mental health advocate but by someone who has experienced depression and suicidal thoughts. As a person who has experienced bouts of depression because of loss of loved ones and suicidal thoughts because of the inability to find hope I write this to encourage others to be free, to be vocal and to seek the help that is needed from a professional if necessary.

To all families, professionals, clergy and everyone who decides to pick this book up to read my hope and prayer is that this book will help you help others and in turn be a guide to help bring further awareness for those who are living with mental illness.

"It is our duty as a people and community to help **#silencethestigma** of mental illness, because you never know when you or someone close to you will have an experience that will cause their mental health to lapse." – L. Marie

This book is dedicated to my vibrant aunt who did not have the opportunity to read this book before it was finished. As she made an impact on this earth with helping families, I hope by telling a very small portion of her story it will continue to help make a difference in the lives of others.

Table of Contents

Have the Conversation

Having the conversation with someone you love about their mental health can be a challenging one. Sometimes you are not ready for what you might hear and other times the person is not ready to talk because they are not prepared for what may come next. Either way it is important to have the conversation as it is the beginning to providing the support that is needed for the person you care about.

What is Mental Illness

Mental illness is a medical disorder that affects people throughout the world. It is nothing to be ashamed of just as asthma, cancer, diabetes and other medical disorders it is something that can be treated. Mental illnesses are health conditions involving changes in emotions, thinking or behavior (or a combination of these).1 Statics show that one in five (19 %) U.S. adults experience some form of mental illness, one in twenty-four (4.1%) has a serious mental illness and one in twelve (8.5%) has a diagnosable substance use disorder.

Look at is this way for every five people you know they have experienced some form of mental illness. That is a high percentage of people and many of them do not have the conversation about what is going on with them because they are ashamed, and they do not want people to look at them different. If someone was diagnosed with kidney disease and never told their love ones or sought treatment what would happen to them? What type of life would they live? I can tell you, not a good one. They would be sick all of the time and in the hospital probably more times than not and if they never received the care they needed they could die.

So, have the conversation and use the information in this book to help better support someone who has a mental illness.

The Culture Says "NO"

Many reasons people don't get help because they were raised not to because the culture said, "it's not what we do." I will not get a lot of likes for this one and that is okay but the culture is wrong and everyone no matter origin needs help and because we cannot do anything alone it is important that we are sensitive to the culture but help break the stigma associated with mental health so people can begin to not only have the conversation within the different cultures but also begin the treatment that is needed.

I cannot speak on every culture and will not attempt to do so, but from working in the mental health field for over fourteen years it has allowed me to see many things. One of the saddest to see is a person who is hurting but will not seek treatment because they are afraid of what their family will say and or how they might embarrass their family because they were taught to leave personal issues within their home and or to just pray about it. And even though talking with your family can be a helpful tool as well as praying, professional help was created to work in conjunction with these other tools.

A suggestion for anyone who is struggling to have the conversation because of your beliefs and upbringing, find a professional with whom you will feel comfortable and that will understand your hesitation because they too are from the same cultural background.

Listen to What Your Loved One Has to Say

What's the most important part of a conversation? I am glad you asked, it is listening for understanding and not for replying. Many times, we do not have on our listening ears and this can cause more confusion and frustration that not. When someone you love initiates the conversation concerning their mental health as we tell our children put on your listening ears so you can hear what they are communicating to you.

Do not assume they are making it up, do not assume they are seeking attention, and do not assume that you know what they are feeling or what they are going through. Even if you believe they are making it up (having a psychosomatic episode, when a person has physical symptoms because of mental conflicts and unresolved problems) be that support until they are able to figure out what is going on with them. When you put on your ears to listen for understanding you become a better support to help them continue to the process of sharing and healing.

Oh yeah, one more thing be sure to check your facial expressions and body language as these indicators will speak louder than any words you can ever speak out of your mouth. A shift in your body posture, an eye rolled, looking away at your phone without saying excuse me, and or looking uninterested in what they have to say can prevent them from continuing the conversation. All the things that are important to you when you are sharing something of concern apply that and then some in order to be present and in the moment with the person you love.

Allow Them to go at Their Own Pace

Your loved one has your ear and you want to ask a lot of questions and or you want to know everything that is going on and that is okay but allow them to tell you in their own timing. Timing is everything and it felt rushed or pressured this can cause one to shut down and question your motives for wanting to know some much. Give them the space and time to come to you on their own terms. When they come to you remember conversation not debate is what is needed for them to process what is going on with them.

Debating will cause them to further shut down and can make them feel like you want to label them like everyone else. If they have not fully processed what is going on, that is okay because with your listening to them it is helping build the trust and rapport that will be needed down the line. They are a glass house, fragile and anything can cause them to break. As a person from the outside looking in you see things one way and as them being the person on in the inside looking out, they see it another. You can both be right but being right will not help with healing nor will it provide them support. Be the safe space they need.

"One small crack does not mean that you are broken, it means that you were put to the test and you didn't fall apart." – Linda Poindexter

2.

Gather Understanding

Don't Judge

Judgement comes from our own bias and whether it is meant or not can cause someone you love to shut down if they believe you are judging them for sharing what is going on with them. What does judgment look like anyway? Well, it can be a combination of things, but I will list a few to help you be aware and more conscious of your actions. Here are some judging behaviors: making fun of someone, thinking they are seeking attention, avoidance (not spending time and or ignoring their calls/texts), having negative thoughts, and using language that can hurt their feelings. We often use the word "crazy" when joking around but have to condition ourselves to not use this word because it can be offensive and hurt the person we love unknowingly.

Did you know judging is one of the main reasons many people who have a mental illness do not come forward and ask for help. It is the main cause why people isolate, self-mutilate and why many parents, spouses, and or loved one say they never seen it coming. When a person feels or believes they are being judged it causes them to feel stigmatized and it causes them to become silent. Silence is not the answer and the only thing that should be silenced is the stigma associated with having a mental health disorder.

Think about it this way, when was the last time you felt judge? What thoughts went through your head about the people who mattered to you the most? I don't know the situation, but you do and remember how isolated and alone you felt because of this judgement; now consider how your love one feels when they are ashamed to talk about something they have no control over. Having a mental illness is a sign that your mental health needs attending to.

Anytime you think about judging I want you to remember what it felt like and not judge the person who is asking for help but provide them the support that you needed when you had your experience.

Educate Yourself on What You Just Heard

The information you just received may have blown your mind and you are not sure how to process it. Well, the good about the age we live in is that we have more information and resources out our fingertips than the generations before us. Some of it is vital and some of it is not, so let's focus on the vital information.

The person you love has informed you they have been going thru some difficult times and they have not been feeling like themselves, so they went to talk with someone, and they have been given an answer to their problem. What they have shared with you is something you do not understand and some of the times they do not either, so they are looking for you to support them. How do you do that? Glad you asked! We begin by educating ourselves, the same way you would educate yourself if a loved one was diagnosed with kidney disease or heart failure, you put forth the same effort and educate yourself on the information you have received.

Research their diagnosis, ask if you can attend a session with them, ask if it is okay for you to speak with their service provider (therapist, psychologist, psychiatrist, etc), and if nothing else ask them what it means to them to have been given this information. Any form of information can be overwhelming but when you don't understand it, it can become frightening and can have adverse reactions. Your support with helping them understand what it they are going through and will have to go through can make it a little easier as they know from the beginning they are not alone.

Understand education goes beyond a book, an article, or information obtained from the internet and sometimes information from the internet can cause more harm than good. The education that is needed will involve a collective of the above mentioned items as well as speaking with professionals who have worked with others facing the same illness including those who are living healthy productive lives. Just as with a medical diagnosis a mental illness requires different forms of treatment and sometimes this includes medication.

Educate Yourself on Their Medications (if it applies)

In educating yourself to be a better support for your love one they may have told you that they have to take medication as a part of their treatment. With this you want to find out what medication(s) they are taking, the dosage, how many times they have to take it, and for how long. You want to inquire if this is a long term part of treatment or temporary, will their provider consider increasing the dosage if it is no longer beneficial and it is always good to know what the side effects of a medication are so the individual will know if this is something they are experiencing. Side effects can be a part of taking medications and when people don't like the way the medication is making them feel they will stop taking it instead of speaking with their provider about other options and changing their dosage. When they share this with you encourage them to call their prescriber and or schedule an appointment and even suggest going with them again providing them the support they need but may not know how to ask for. Education is not only essential for the person with the mental illness, but it is essential to those that have promised to be a part of the support net.

As a supporter the more you understand can allow your love one to be empowered so they will understand how every step of their treatment plays into their healing. When we are misinformed or lack the knowledge that is needed, we can say and do things that are not helpful to the people we care for. These attitudes of unawareness can prevent our love ones from receiving treatment and in turn cause a downward spiral; we want them to get better and stay that way. A friendly reminder ensures they continue to take their medication even if they begin to feel better, if they stop taking their medications it can cause them to slip back into old behaviors and in turn have to start fresh with this part of treatment.

Feeling better is great and allows them to know the treatment is working, but if they would like to stop with the medication strongly and firmly suggest they speak with their provider so they can effectively come up with a plan that will allow them to continue treatment in a beneficial way.

Learn About Their Diagnosis and Treatment Options

How many of you have been given a medical diagnosis or had a love one receive one? The first thing you do is ask questions, like what does this mean, what lifestyle changes are needed, can this be reverse, etc. Well, the same applies when you have a loved one diagnosed with depression, anxiety, bipolar, schizophrenia, oppositional defiant disorder (ODD), and or attention-deficit/hyperactivity disorder (ADHD). I could list more, but the point here is we cannot base what we see in movies, television or what someone heard be the basis of the information we have to provide the support that is needed for someone we care about. We have to understand what it means to have this disorder/diagnosis, what are the symptoms associated with it and what is the appropriate level of treatment that can be provided to help with ensuring the healing that is needed can take place.

If someone has asthma, they will not follow the same treatment regimen as someone who has a heart disease. I know you are thinking why I continue to reference medical disorders, well because I want you to understand just as we focus on our physical health we have to put just as much attention and effort into our mental health. The way you begin to make changes in order for your physical health to be intact is just as important for you to put in the same effort to ensure you and your loved one's mental health is intact. Small changes such as more or less sleep, exercise, changing eating habits, who we hang around and how we maintain relationships can all help with getting better not just physical but our emotional, physical, and spiritual (holistic healing). We cannot focus on one area of health and not all.

"Healing takes time and asking for help is a courageous step."

– Mariska Hargitay

3.

Provide Support

Accept the Diagnosis

Denial is the easy part of life, it is not accepting the realities of our life. This provides people the ability to control the narrative and denial is associated with the beliefs one has about what mental illness is. Your acceptance of their diagnosis will help your love one begin to accept it as well. The beginning journey will not be an easy one because for them acceptance will mean there is a problem and they are not ready to address this problem. By you accepting their diagnosis and educating yourself on what it means to have their symptoms, what is required for treatment and be vocal about how you will support them it can help them come around to accepting their diagnosis as well. No one wants to feel or seem like an outcast and for this reason many people are in denial about what is happening with them even after they have sought help.

Acceptance is not judgement, but it is love, support, help, and guidance. Why, did I add this because I have seen families torn apart because they have the acceptance piece down, but they forget the support. They forget that just because they have accepted the changes that have happened their loved ones have not. Imagine being "normal" and then you begin to notice changes with your body that are not explainable, only to find out that you have to live with a change that most people find uncomfortable because they don't understand. Others have accepted this, but you are still trying to process it all, well this is exactly how your family member feels. They are trying to process it and some days it will make sense but on other days it will not. On the days where it doesn't, help them understand as you are learning so you can help be sure to involve them in the process, this makes it easier for your and them. Love, support, comfort, not judgment; Be their safe space!

It is important to remind the person how much you love them, how you will help them adjust to their new normal, how you will be an advocate for them if it is needed, and how you will always be there as a support for them.

With acceptance of the diagnosis it provides a different level of support which can include you helping make appointments, attending appointments with them, and or helping with ensuring they take their medications as prescribed. When they are in denial, they will remember your kind words and gestures which will help them reach out for and accept your help. Denying the diagnosis will not change their behaviors, symptoms or mental illness, but acceptance will help get them on the path to healing.

Have Realistic Expectations

Recovery like with anything will take time and just as a road has bumps, turns, and straight ways so does someone on the road to healing with mental illness. Even when you see their symptoms, moods and or behaviors changing provide the support needed in that space because anything can happen that can cause a setback. In the moments when setbacks happen reiterate your love, support, encouragement, and acceptance of what is going on with them. A setback for your love one is more frustrating to them than it will ever be to you. There will be moments of confusion for you and them, during those times encourage an extra appointment with their therapist, utilize the tools that have been given to help them, and be the ear that is needed. They already feel judged by those outside of their support net they do not need the judgement from you.

A setback can cause one to have to be hospitalized and that is okay, if this happens with your love one offer to go with them so they don't feel alone during this process. Hospitalization is not a scare tactic, it is not a scare straight program, and it is not a form of punishment. When someone has to go to the hospital it is because they are sick and need help. This help can include medication adjustment, a change in treatment, a change in service provider and or a change in the support that is being provided. I have seen too many families use hospitalization as a way to scare a love one to "get straight" but this does not help but can cause them to shut down and shut you out when they feel threaten for expressing their thoughts and emotions. Hospitalization is a form of treatment and sometimes multiple visits is what is needed in order to get the right treatment in place.

Some things are not preventable and whatever they need from you to help get them back on track do that. Realistic expectations will help them understand the ups and downs of treatment and because they have your support, they will get through this like they have with other setbacks in their life.

I offer this story as a way to help you understand that realistic expectations will not only help you but the person you care about. Working in an inpatient treatment facility you see a lot of things and encounter families from different walks of life. You do your best as a provider to meet the needs of all the families and patients you come in contact with but there are times when this is not the case. There was a family whose child was admitted to the facility because of aggressive behaviors towards themselves and others. The family had been through this before with their child being hospitalized but was unsure of what caused this episode. The identified patient was adamant about harming themselves and threaten to harm anyone that they thought would get in their way to stop them. They were attending sessions as scheduled and as reported was taking their medication as recommended. However, they were agitated all the time, not eating and having trouble sleeping; these were new symptoms for their family, and they were concerned about the wellbeing of the other children because this child was escalating. Long story short, this patient needed a change in their medication to help with their changed behaviors and was able to discover there was some trauma that had taken place in this patients life that they had not talked about and was triggered by something they had seen on television. The family was unaware of this trauma as this child was adopted, and it happened before the child became to be a part of this family.

Understand you may not know everything about your love one and realize there are things that happen to people that they will never talk about. If you notice a change in behavior consider that something could have happened that triggered this and what you thought recovery to look like will be different from what it really is. As it is stated for every action there is a reaction (this can be good or bad).

Recognizing Triggers

Do you know what triggers you when you become upset? What is the thing(s) that cause you to go over the edge? Many people don't know and because of it have found themselves in some really uncomfortable situations. Well, if you were not able to identify your triggers can you imagine what it is like for someone to have a mental health crisis because they do not know their triggers. Helping your love ones identify their triggers can be helpful when they are experiencing a crisis.

There was a client I used to work with, and they had a hard time controlling their anger. When they became upset, they would ask not to be touched and it was important that you gave them at least five minutes to themselves before you started a conversation with them. These things were important as if you touched them or talked to them before they were ready this would trigger them and cause them to become more irritable and agitated. When they did not receive the support that was needed it was hard to calm them down, however, because there was a plan in place this was helpful to control the outburst and lessen the behavior from becoming violent. Knowing someone's triggers can help prevent a mental health crisis and prevent your love one from being hospitalized.

Another individual had a hard time with anxiety and for the most part did not know what triggered them, they knew when they felt this way they needed to get away from others as they had not expressed to many, they suffered from panic attacks. While at work one day this person begins to experience heavy breathing, sweaty hands, and became overwhelmed with emotions. Nothing had happened in the moment and they did not know what to do or how to handle this which made the panic attack worse because they were afraid to ask for a moment to themselves to get their thoughts together. A question was asked, what triggered this? What were you doing right before this happened? What tools do you have in place to help you when you experience this again at work? They took these questions and realized that writing helps them relieve their anxiety and they identified a support at work to help them get through when they are having a time.

The anniversary of a loss (spouse, parent, child, job, house, etc.) can be the trigger for someone. The smell of a significant other or food can be a trigger also. If someone feels embarrassed or feel like they are being made fun of this can trigger behaviors. We all have triggers, but it is important we are able to identify and help our loved ones identify what triggers them to help reduce the chance of a mental health crisis taking place. Once we have identified the trigger(s) it is also important to have tools in place to help when they are triggered. Tools to help a loved one is a like a tool kit you keep at home for when an emergency happens or when things need to be tightened around the house. It is the same concept having the right tools can help in an emergency or help tighten up situations when they begin to fall apart!

Offer to Pray with Them

Prayer is an essential part of some people's lives and it is what gives them hope that everything is going to be okay. It is open communication with God and sometimes when people are in crisis or find themselves spiraling, they cannot find the strength to pray but need those who are a part of their support net to pray for them and with them. When providing support, ask your loved one is it okay for you to pray with them. Find out what is troubling them and pray with them on that matter. The power of pray can help ease their anxiety, can provide them with peace, and help restore their confidence that everything is going to be okay.

If they have the strength to allow them to lead the prayer, this reassures their power and gives them the opportunity to speak those things that are not as if they were, and it gives them the authority to reclaim who they are in God. Having authority and control over important parts of their life is more important than you will ever know. Belief in God, prayer and treatment can make a major difference in the person you love life so support them. As stated throughout, treatment plans are different for everyone and so are the tools that are in their kits. If prayer is a part of their treatment and is a tool, they need to use often support them in that!

Remember support is different for us all, so support them in the way they need it and not the way you think support should look like.

"I cannot stand the words "Get over it." All of us are under such pressure to put our problems in the past tense. Slow

down. Don't allow other to hurry your healing. It is a process, one that may take years, occasionally, even a lifetime- and that's OK."

– Beau Taplin

Insert from Counseling Psychologist Esther Schmidt

As a Counselling Psychologist I work with clients who experience a variety of mental illness and often times whose family members and friends do not know how to help the individual. When working with a client I know that more often than not I am also working to provide educational information and supports as much as possible to their friends and family members. Often times people are at a loss of where to even start or how to help a loved one when they are struggling or in the midst of their illness.

First and foremost, it is important to have a conversation with the person that is experiencing mental illness. Having open dialogue opens up the communication lines and allows family members to begin to understand the individual more. One of the things that I have found has been key in helping a loved one with mental illness is by starting open dialogue about the mental illness and how the individual themselves is doing. This can help to understand what they are going through but also help them know that you are interested in hearing more about what they are dealing with. It allows them to know that you are open to having a conversation with them. This opens up the opportunity for future conversations. The key point is to not let the individual suffer in silence. Creating spaces to have conversations has been monumental in helping individuals with mental illness feel connected to those in their support circle. This in turn allows them to feel supported and cared for.

On top of all of the above having an open conversation leads to being able to gather a better awareness and understanding on what the individual is currently going through and suffering with.

Gathering information and educating yourself can be huge in being able to be supportive of your loved one. This allows you to gather appropriate information that you need. Gaining an understanding is helpful to your loved one. Often times people with mental illness find it difficult to explain themselves over and over again. To top that off it can be difficult for them to express how they are feeling. Gathering information and educating yourself helps you significantly be able to begin to understand the effects that the mental illness may have on your loved one. It also gives you the proper awareness to be able to know how to step in and help them when needed. It allows you to begin to recognize some patterns quicker and helps identify triggers as well. I always encourage people to do research and educate themselves. Education can go a long way in supporting your loved one or friend. Along with this it is also so important to not come across as the savior. The idea behind learning more and gathering an understanding is to be able to support the individual. The last thing the person needs is someone who is trying to "fix them." The idea is to support them in what they are going through rather than to try and fix something.

The idea here is not about "fixing" anything but rather about supporting the individual while they are in the processes of healing and working through things with their therapist. Your job is not about being a therapist to them - they likely already have one. Your role is to be supportive to the individual and their needs. By doing this the individual will feel supported and calm in the processes. Fixing only ends up giving you exhaustion and created a barrier between you and the loved one.

Providing support may look different for each individual. Often times when I am talking to clients and ask them how friends and family can support them, I hear a variety of different things. One of the main things that I hear is just listening to them and trying to understand. Most of the time the loved one does not expect you to fully understand what they are experiencing or going through. But making an effort to learn more, ask them questions, and being there for them can go a long way.

A key component in supporting a loved one is to provide them with hope. Often times individuals who are in the midst of mental illness often find it difficult to see the light at the end of the tunnel or to find hope in the midst of their despair. Providing hope is a foundational part of your role as a loved one. It allows you to bring that glimpse of hope to them.

As a therapist I see firsthand how having open conversations, gathering understanding, providing support, asking questions, and providing them with hope can make a world of a difference in the therapeutic process as well as in the individual feeling cared for, supported, heard, and known.

Every person has a longing to belong, a longing to be known, and a longing to be heard. When you approach each encounter with individuals in this manner you find yourself being able to have empathy for others. It allows you to have more awareness for the people in your life that may be suffering. Always remember that it is good to have open conversations.

"Sometimes self-care is exercise and eating right. Sometimes it's spending time with loved ones or taking a nap. And sometimes it's watching an entire season of TV in one weekend while you lounge around in your pajamas. Whatever soothes your soul."

– Nanea Hoffman

4.

Ask Questions but Don't Pry

Find Out What It's Like to Live with Their Symptoms

A physical illness can affect the way your body feels and at times prevent you from doing anything enjoyable because your body does not have the strength. With a mental illness it can be the same except your brain does not have the energy and in turn affects your thoughts, emotions and behaviors. So, ask the right questions to help you better understand the symptoms they are experiencing. Here is a list of questions that can be helpful in better understanding your loved one's symptoms:

1. "Can you help me understand what it's like living with your condition?"
2. "How has living with this condition shaped who you are today?"
3. "Is there anything you need from me or something I can do to help you?"
4. "How can I support you- can I listen to you, leave you alone, pray with you, give you a hug?"
5. "Can we do something together?"

This is not an extensive list, but it is a place to help get started and or continue the conversation with someone you love to better understand what it is they are going through. Just like a person with the flu the symptoms can look different from person to person, but here are some symptoms to help you recognize change in behaviors. Again, this is not an extensive list just an idea of what it could look like, always talk with someone before making assumptions about what you think is or is not going on:

- Feeling sad or down
- Excessive fears or worries
- Extreme feelings of guilt
- Withdrawal from family, friends, and enjoyed activities
- Major changes in eating or sleeping habits
- Excessive anger, irritability, hostility, and violence
- Thoughts of self-harm
- Detached from reality (delusions), paranoia or hallucinations

As suggested throughout this book communication is key and will help bring clarity to things that we see in the people we love. It is important that if the person denies these behaviors, but you recognize them that you ask them about any changes that has happened in their life that you are unaware of. Changes in environment and home life can cause these symptoms to arise so be sensitive to what you are asking and the tone with which you use, this can help continue dialogue or cause the person to shut down.

Ensure the Support Net is Strong

Support is a major part of treatment for someone with mental illness and is something that cannot be stressed enough. While I was in grad school, we discussed support and what it meant to us. My professor provided us with a picture of a net and told us to write down the people who we consider our support. The thought here is a net can bring in a lot of fish and so it is considered to be strong and just as a net is strong to hold those fish so should your support system. Your support net should be strong enough to hold you and bring you in when the time is needed. I encourage you to write down who you would put in your net of support and then ask the person you are supporting to write down their net of support. Your support might be more than theirs and vice versa, but it is imperative that you help them identify the people who can catch them and hold them in times of need. It is essential to have the numbers of these people in the event something happens, and if you are not available to be there for your love one they will have an alternate option. Identifying these people can help add to your net of support and allow you to know that you are not doing this alone.

Check In

Weekly and or daily check ins can make the difference of how a person feels and or thrives in their healing. We are living in times where you can send someone a text as a form of checking in and this lets them know they were on your mind. Many of us have busy schedules but let's not become too busy with life that we forget to check on the people who we say matter to us most.

Now, a text may not always be the answer and there will be times you need to pick up the phone and hear their voice to make sure they are actually okay. As we all know when you don't want people to know we are going through we tend to say whatever is needed through text and are thankful the person did not call because they could hear we are not doing well. One thing better than text and a phone call is video chat which is now available on every smartphone.

Seeing someone is better than hearing their voice and reading words on a screen. This allows you to look into someone's eyes and truly connect with them. The benefit of having video chat is when you don't live in the same state, city or country you still have the ability to see those we care about. Growing up we can only imagine doing this, depending on when you grew up, we had the "Jetsons" and some of us had "Kim Possible" to give us a glimpse of what this would look like. As excited as we were with having this, now that it is available we don't use it as often as we should.

There are so many ways to check in now that even Facebook and Instagram allows you to call or video with someone from your phone or computer. We no longer have an excuse of why we cannot be there for those who matter. Hey, if you want there is still the old fashion way of writing a letter (shrugs shoulders).

What I am saying is no matter the form of checking in be like the Nike slogan and JUST DO IT!

Checking in is different for us all and so find out what works best for the person you are supporting.

Find Out How You Can Support Them

Support is a big part of treatment and something that is needed by all people with or without a mental illness. But what we have to know and remember support does not look the same for everyone. Some people prefer being in the presence of others, some want conversation, others want to go out, some want to stay in, and others well the list can go on, but you get what I am saying. What I am encouraging you to do is provide them with the support they need and not the support you think they need. When you ask about what support is needed it allows them to be empowered and a part of their treatment options. Ensure what they are asking is something that is reasonable and doable, and at times ask if it is okay to make suggestions. But do not force your meaning of support on them because this will show them you were not listening to hear their needs, but you were listening to provide them with what you thought they wanted and or needed to hear. So, when you ask them how you can support them listen to what they are asking and don't allow it to be the last time you ask because their needs will change within the path of their illness.

"Anything that's human is mentionable, and anything that is mentionable can be more manageable. When we can talk about our feelings, they become less overwhelming, less upsetting, and less scary." – Fred Rogers

5.

Provide Them with Hope

Provide Healthy Distractions

A mental illness does not define who a person is, but it is a part of their everyday journey. For this reason, you should encourage them to continue to engage in their normal healthy activities. If they play an instrument, are in band, choir, group, if they write, are athletic or whatever their healthy coping skill of life is encourage them to continue to do those things. Maintaining a "normal" life and routine is also a part of healthy healing and treatment.

If they were not doing anything before learning about their mental illness than help them find something they like and suggest that you and some of their other friends/family do it as a group. Keeping them active and participating in everyday life activities will help them not focus on their illness, but on living a healthy full life. It will allow their mind to stay active, help balance their emotions, and their behaviors. When you are sick most of the time all you want to do is be still, but we know this is not good for the body. And if you didn't know, it has been studied that sitting still, laying down, and not being active is the leading cause to many other illnesses. Because we don't want them to get worse, we want to encourage constant movement and for them to be active.

Take them to a concert, karaoke night, listen to jazz, a comedy show, or whatever they find entertaining. Allow them to pick and when or if they cannot think of anything then you help them look up something that can spark their interest. Healthy distractions help normalize life and exposes them to things they did not know they were interested in.

Often times a healthy distraction does not always have to involve arts and or recreational activities. A healthy distraction can be political, religious, and or being more involved in their community. Whatever, the healthy distraction is please provide them with the support that is needed.

Be an Advocate with and For Them

What does it mean to be an advocate? Well, let me start with what an advocate is not. An advocate is not someone who is perfect and who has never expressed a bad day or felt like giving up. They are not people who have don't have a mental illness nor are they people who have never had a mental health crisis. A mental health advocate is not perfect, but they are perfect in that they find the strength to give a voice for people like them and for people who they understand cannot find their voice yet even though the seek daily to show self-care and support for others.

An advocate is someone who provides a voice to help bring awareness to something that is going on within their communities. Being an advocate with the person you love helps them tell their journey about what it is like to live with a mental illness and how they are thriving in everyday life. It helps them shed light on how they overcome daily struggles and how their treatment is getting them through allowing them to heal in the proper way. This doesn't mean they don't have struggles, but they have found what is needed to get through these struggles.

You being an advocate separate from your love one still gives them a voice, but it's given from the voice of the supporter. You help educate the community on mental illness and reduce the stigma associated with having a mental health disorder along with bringing awareness to promote change in the behavioral health system. Your voice and actions help become the change agent that is needed within the community. Your support helps break barriers, injustices and makes others aware of how they too can become an advocate for others in their community and within their family.

Talk to Someone You Can Trust

Being an advocate for someone is a great task but sometimes comes with other responsibilities beyond educating the community and bringing awareness. Depending on the diagnosis of your loved one you may have to make some major changes, like become their mental health power of attorney, become their guardian (if it's an adult or a child who has now become an adult), and or have been assigned by the court because this person can longer make sound judgement to handle their affairs. With this continued and or new responsibility you will need to talk with someone you can trust.

Just as you are a part of this person's support net you too will need a separate support net. You will need to have people who can provide you sound advice, can help you look up treatment options, help you process day to day task, and or being that shoulder you need when you are feeling overwhelmed. Being a caretaker no matter the disorder can be a strain and if you do not take care of yourself how effective are you with helping be there for the person you love.

There was a lady whose husband was diagnosed with cancer and she became his full-time caretaker until the day he died. When he passed, she was sad but glad the love of her life was no longer suffering. She had not taken a moment for herself the entire time he was ill because she felt she needed to be by his side every step of the way. The day I met her was the first time she had done something for herself and it was a simple pedicure. We chatted for a while and I provided her some encouraging words and then I allowed her to relax in her moment. She had provided day in and day out care for her husband, she showed up when no one else would or could, she did not miss a beat and you could tell even with the support she had she did not fully lean on them as she did not want to be a burden. In her moment of silence, she had found peace that she had done all she could and that her husband had fought the good fight, but now was at rest and so could she. You could tell the nap she took while getting her pedicure was the first time she actually could sleep without feeling like she would have to jump up and tend to the needs of someone else. She was at peace within herself and had begun the journey of self-care.

I know you are thinking her husband had cancer how is that the same as having a mental illness. Let me bring clarity to this, it can be the same because some people who have a mental illness require constant care to ensure their love one is taking their medications, attending their therapy sessions, exercising, eating right, sleeping right, and doing all the other things that have been created in their Person Centered Plan (PCP). There are treatment facilities but many are not comfortable with putting their loves one in long term care nor do some families have the resources that it takes to ensure around the clock care is provided and so they have to do it themselves.

Here is a personal story that I share with you with permission from my cousin. My aunt who was a vibrant woman, full of life loved traveling, and a giver to her community and family. She began to have a change in her behavior and the family did not know why. She had planned to retire but before making the decision to do so was forced.

When she retired it was as if her health declined (previous diagnosis of congestive heart failure) more and she was diagnosed with early stages of dementia. This rocked our family as this was not the path we saw for her. One of the behaviors that can be experienced with this disorder is aggressive behavior. She had to be hospitalized and during this time had an aggressive episode. When this happens to an individual in order to keep the patient and staff safe, they have to restrain the patient. She was in an unfamiliar place and wanted to go home and be with people and things that were familiar to her; she did not want to be in a strange place, nor did she feel like she belong there. She did not even know she was exhibiting this behavior.

Before her release the disease had progressed and to ensure the appropriate care was in place for her safety and continue progress with adapting to the changes that would come with this disease the assigned social worker had to ensure my aunt had a caretaker to provide around the clock care. This care would include her eating, bathing, taking her medications, and her safety.

Her husband works and was not familiar with the disease or the responsibilities that came with being a caretaker and her children are grown, so what was the family to do? Step up and work together and work the plan that was put into place to ensure the care she needed was received and that is what happened. A home health aide that works with patients with Dementia/Alzheimer's was sent to work with her, friends of the family chipped in, her son, husband and sister created a schedule for the weekends that would work to ensure she would be supported.

Yes, if someone wants help they should put in the effort to ensure they are getting it, but as you can see the choice is not always up to the person who wants or need the help because most of the time they have no control of what is happening to them. For families who have love ones with Dementia/Alzheimer's, level two or three autism, intellectual disability disorder, and or down syndrome to name a few require more attention and support. Whatever role you find yourself in as a supporter of someone with a mental illness be sure you have a person you too can lean on when it is time.

This has been mentioned a few times in this book and that is because it is key to maintaining your mental health, **SELF-CARE** is what is needed to be a support to others!

The Conversation is not Always About Mental Illness
If you were to find out you were sick would you want this to be the only conversation someone had with you? Of course not, you would want people to talk with you about everyday life and to continue to treat you like before they found out you were sick. The same is for someone is who has a mental illness. They don't need to be remined about their daily struggles, as it is something they have to deal with daily.

Earlier we mentioned to ask the person "how can I support you?" this is a question that does not stop but is continuous because with each day and each event someone experiences require different levels of support. To bring it more relatable we are now in a pandemic and everyone no matter class, race, gender, religion, etc. we are all experiencing the same thing, but we are not all experiencing it the same way. For someone who is a recovering addict and or has anxiety, depression, autism, depression, etc. this is rough in a different way. The support they are used to is no longer, the connection of personal interaction with others that is needed for their treatment looks a lot different than it did just a few months ago. How much more support is needed now than before?

So, back to the conversation at hand no the conversation is not always about their mental illness, but it is about their progress with dealing with life on a day to day and situation by situation. It is being supportive, going to dinner, the movies, gallery, and whatever else was done to allow them to live life as normal.

"What mental health needs is more sunlight, more candor, and more unashamed conversations."- Glenn Close

Before the chapters and table of contents began my note to you and your family was my desire and hope of writing this book was to provide families and the community with the tools needed to support their love ones with mental illness. A lot of information has been provided and it will not take at one time but an approach overtime and so does the support that is needed for someone to be successful in their treatment.

"You are not supposed to fit in, so stop trying. Make others fit to you and if they don't it is okay because all things that are special stand out and sometimes, they have to stand alone." – L. Marie

notes

Chapter 1. Have the Conversation

1. https://www.psychiatry.org/patients-families/what-is-mental-illness

resources

NAMI Helpline*
-800-950-6264 or text "NAMI" to 741741 (24/7, confidential free crisis counseling)

National Suicide Prevention Lifeline*
-800-273-TALK (8255); En Español 888-628-9454 (24 hours a day)

Crisis Text Line*
-Text "HELLO" TO 741741 (24 hours a day)

Veterans Crisis Line*
-800-273-TALK (8255) and press 1 (24 hours a day 7 seven days a week)

Disaster Distress Helpline*
-800-985-5990 or text "TalkWithUs" to 66746 (24 hours a day 7 days a week)

SAMHSA's National Helpline*
-800-662-HELP (4357) (24 hours a day 7 days a week; treatment referral and information)

Seize The Awkward*
-Text SEIZE to 741741 (24 hours a day 7 days a week); visit **www.seizetheawkward.com**

This is not an exhaustive list but a small resource guide to help you get started

www.ingramcontent.com/pod-product-compliance
Lightning Source LLC
Chambersburg PA
CBHW070258290326
41930CB00041B/2639